YOGA MUDRA
ORACLE

Yoga Mudra Oracle

Transformative Spiritual Power in Your Hands

EMMA WERTHEIM

This edition published in 2024 by Arcturus Publishing Limited
26/27 Bickels Yard, 151–153 Bermondsey Street,
London SE1 3HA

AD012446US

Printed in China

CONTENTS

CARD MEANINGS cont.

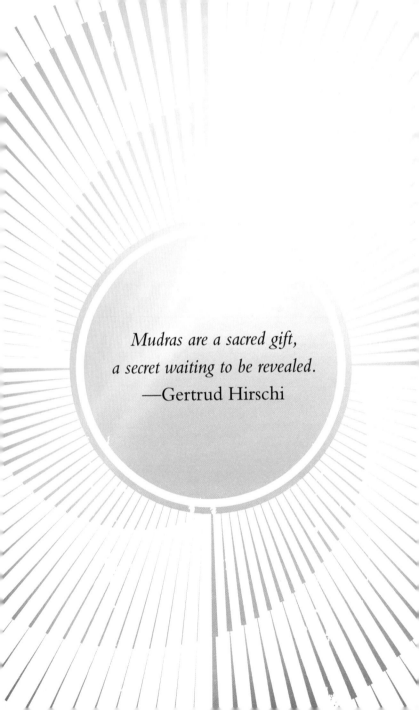

Mudras are a sacred gift,
a secret waiting to be revealed.
—Gertrud Hirschi

INTRODUCTION

The story behind
Yoga Mudra Oracle

Towards the end of my yoga teacher training, my health took a turn. In a world of pain, I found myself unable to do basic *asanas* or even walk at times. I started looking for something I could do that would make me feel better and required only minimal physical exertion.

I had heard about yoga *mudras* involving hand gestures. But aside from *Anjali mudra* (also known as 'prayer pose'), which is performed at the end of most yoga classes, I didn't know much about them. I discovered that the word *mudra* has Sanskrit origins translating to "seal," "mark," or "gesture," and that mudras can involve not just the hands but other parts of the body. I learned that the term *Hasta mudras* refers specifically to yogic hand postures, which are the focus of *Yoga Mudra Oracle*.

For as long as I can remember, I've been aware of people's hands as much as their faces. For me, hands tell a lot about a person. I never gave it much thought, however, until late in 2016, when I delved deeper into mudras and their healing potential. It was a rabbit hole I dived down; I absorbed as much information as possible and read every book I could find.

To my surprise, I discovered there is a mudra to help with pretty much everything—from detoxifying to building immunity or healing earache. There are also more spiritual postures for connecting with cosmic energy and receiving divine guidance. Mudras are multipurpose and have multifaceted benefits.

I also realized that for more than 25 years, without knowing it, I had been using *Dhyana mudra*—the yogic hand posture of meditation—as part of my daily meditative practice. Yes, mudras can find you! Reflecting on this, I have come to understand that my hands evoke my peaceful state as a natural expression of what is happening in my body.

I'm surprised how rarely mudras are practiced in yoga classes. If you have stumbled across this deck, maybe it is for a reason. Perhaps things are about to change as more and more people become aware of the magical world of mudras and their transformational potential.

It is my heart's wish that—like me—you might discover how mudras can change your life on a profound level. I am certain they will support you, whatever stage of your journey you're at. They are an easy, efficient and accessible way to reap the benefits of yoga in your own time and space.

Of course, I'm not recommending you skip your yoga classes! I'm just saying that mudras can be of immediate benefit to you on many levels. The more you work with them, the more easily you will be able to sense and experience a vibrational shift in your body.

In my own personal work, I have come to believe mudras have a sun-like quality. They have an energy that nurtures lifeforce—also known as *prana* or *chi*—to be pure and strong. Yet they are potent too—mystically and subtly supporting life on Earth.

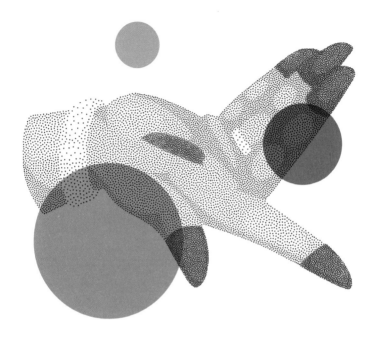

WELCOME TO *YOGA MUDRA ORACLE*

The birth of *Yoga Mudra Oracle* has been a gradual process, seeded mysteriously over the years in a way that felt destined. Mudras are an expression of ancient spirituality. They have been practiced for thousands of years, passed down by enlightened yoga masters (seers) as a gift to us. They hold great mystery and power.

Mudras evoke our hidden inner resources—helping us unite with a universal, cosmic energy. By taking a yoga mudra gesture with our hands and grounding ourselves in the conscious breath, we simply and powerfully 'seal' a specific flow of energy in the body. In turn, this creates a pranic (energy) circuit or resonance within us. This supports us in accessing deeper intuition and invites our physical body to heal. Ultimately, we open ourselves to universal energy and the influence of the Divine, which can give rise to elevated states of consciousness.

Yoga Mudra Oracle celebrates the power and beauty of mudras and what they allow us to experience.

Similar to foot reflexology, all areas of the hands are thought to connect to corresponding organs, glands, nerves, and meridians throughout the body. Mudras also incorporate aspects of palmistry, Ayurveda, acupressure, and the Chinese Five Elements philosophy.

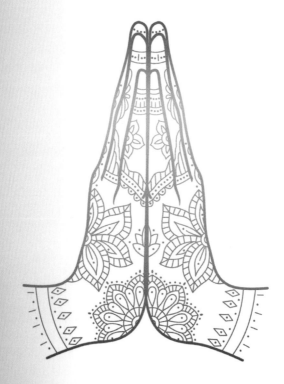

Yoga mudras have been recognized in traditions such as Buddhism and Hinduism. *Jnana mudra* appears in depictions of Hindu deities, and the Buddhist name for this same posture is *Vitarka mudra*. Byzantine icons also show Christ using various mudras. One of the best-known mudras in yoga is *Anjali*, or 'prayer pose' (also referred to as *Namaskar mudra*). Present in both Eastern and Western cultures, this posture is associated with humility, divine offering, reverence, salutation and innermost wishes. From simple, easily available hand gestures, the most profound feelings and experiences can emerge.

Mudras can be compared to slow-release medicine. Consistent exploration and practice bring about holistic renewal, with many scientific studies confirming this. When healing occurs, you experience the world around you in a new and different way.

There are several hundred hand mudras identified in the yogic tradition. *Yoga Mudra Oracle* offers 44 of these, each depicting a single mudra hand gesture. As a selection from the wider spectrum, the mudras of *Yoga Mudra Oracle* express the great esoteric principle that every part is a reflection of the whole— "As above, so below."

The deck also includes some non-traditional, "intuited" yoga mudras. These help us open to higher guidance. In a similar way, readers may wish to explore and create their own mudras when working with the deck.

All mudras have been chosen for their balancing, healing and enlightening qualities. Each one is a practice in its own right, which features in the guidance provided for each card. The mudras and their messages can be used to expand your yoga or meditative practice, or for quick advice in the moment. The cards can also be consulted with or without practising the mudras. Even just meditating on the mudra and its meaning can be of benefit.

Yoga Mudra Oracle has been assembled with great love and care. To preserve its purity, the creative development process has been kept free of the ordinary self as much as possible. We hope you feel this too, as you explore its possibilities.

Yoga is not exclusively aligned with any one religion. Similarly, this oracle deck is rooted in spirituality, while honouring and respecting all traditions, backgrounds and practices. It is a fusion of philosophies, esoteric ideals, and practices with ancient yogic principles.

You will encounter words such as: "divine", "God", "femininity", "mother", "father", "cosmos", "universe" and "spirit". You may exchange any of these for words or concepts for those compatible with your own belief system.

Most importantly, you are encouraged to sense and feel, entering into the energy of the words and ideas. After all, the "word" is simply a tool to communicate a particular vibration.

Allow *Yoga Mudra Oracle* to take you on a journey of self-discovery – revealing gems of wisdom and flashes of insight, shedding light on who you are and your calling in this lifetime. As you ponder the card meanings and their associated mudra poses, may you connect to an inner self that transcends space and time, putting you in touch with an expanded vision of your life and soul purpose.

By activating each card's guidance, you allow the mudras to manifest, flowing into your everyday life and helping your heartfelt truths become a reality. You don't need to sit on a mountaintop, in an isolated cave or attend a sweaty, 120-minute Bikram yoga class! You may be sitting in your car at traffic lights, watching television or standing in a crowded shopping mall when you take a mudra pose and change your day for the better.

Mudras are accessible and safe for everyone! They can be practiced anywhere, by anyone, at any time.

Please note: *mudras should not replace medical advice or expertise—they work best as supplementary support on your healing journey.*

How to prepare your hands for mudras

The more you work with mudras, the more your hands will become supple and fall easily into the poses. At first, this might feel difficult or challenging. Don't worry, it gets easier.

To prepare, first become aware of your breath deepening into your belly. Feel your rhythm change as your body slows. Take a deep breath. Clap your hands together firmly three times, then exhale. Next, with your hands pressed full length against each other, rub them together for 60 seconds. Stop once they are warm.

You are now ready to begin practising mudras.

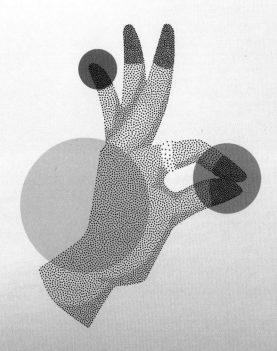

How long do I hold the mudra?

Hold each mudra for at least three conscious breaths when working with the deck. However, if you wish to extend the session, anywhere between five and 45 minutes is optimal. You can practice mudras throughout the day—e.g. in 15-minute intervals, three times a day. Explore the possibilities and find your own way. You may wish to include mudras in your meditation practice or as part of a card reading. Try different ways of integrating them into your day-to-day life.

When you become more familiar with mudras and their benefits, you may choose to work with one or several of them for a few days or even longer, depending on your desired outcome. For example, *Chonmukha Mukha mudra* strengthens the immune system. If you pull this card when you're feeling run down, you might work with it for several days or even weeks until you feel stronger.

Again, there is nothing wrong with taking a mudra pose while stationary at the wheel in traffic, waiting in various situations, in gatherings, while travelling or walking. *Jnana mudra*, for example, helps you feel grounded and energetically protected. You might find it beneficial in large crowds or when your energy is scattered.

Expand your understanding by incorporating mudras into your day. Use the postures you find most supportive or others you may intuitively receive as "gifts" through your work with the deck.

Don't be disheartened by fatigue when you start working with *Yoga Mudra Oracle*. It is a sign that the process has begun. In time, the tiredness will shift. You may find some mudras work almost instantly for you, while others have a more subtle influence. Discover what suits you best.

Always remember to relax your shoulders when working with mudras. Be patient, explore, play and experiment. Let mudras show you the way!

What if a mudra doesn't resonate with me?

Don't use it. But always give it a chance. Even if it hasn't worked for you before, it might be the mudra you need right now.

What if my hands can't make the shapes of the mudras?

Don't be concerned. Make sure you warm up your hands properly before trying the mudra. The more you work with it, the more you develop muscle memory and the easier it gets. If it's too difficult, however, hold it for as long as is comfortable—then give your hands a rest. If all else fails, meditate on the mudra shape and the guidance provided.

Why are intuited/non-traditional mudras included?

Yoga Mudra Oracle combines traditional yoga mudras and a small selection of non-traditional or "intuited" mudras. These intuited mudras have a place in this deck, with their ability to arouse a particular feeling or experience.

If you feel the impulse to create or "make up" a non-traditional mudra, don't hesitate. Also, be sure to share it on social media so others can try it too! Also, if you have the urge to go into a "moving mudra"—by adding dynamic movement—feel free to do that. Conversely, if you feel resistance to using the mudra associated with one of the cards in the deck, it's okay not to use it. The card message may be sufficient itself, or the mudra might be adequate on its own.

What does each card include?

Each card message provides guidance in the following format:

Title: the traditional name of the mudra.

Subtitle: a one-line summary of the mudra's guidance.

Key themes: the core ideas or symbols associated with the mudra.

Main message: in-depth guidance related to the mudra.

Mudra: how to physically practice the mudra.

Affirmation: a short, affirmative statement to help you integrate the mudra's message into your life. It can be spoken aloud or observed silently.

All methods are up to you and quite acceptable. Whatever way you use *Yoga Mudra Oracle*, it will be an enriching experience.

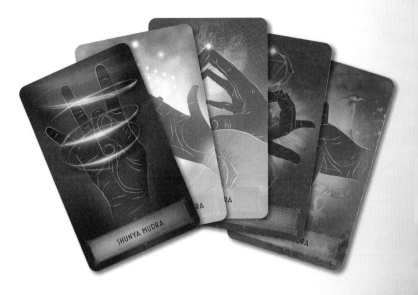

Can I work with just the guidance and not the mudras, or vice versa?

Each mudra hand gesture allows you to integrate the card's message more deeply on a physical and cellular level and open your consciousness to another reality. However, it's not necessary to perform the gesture if you're time-poor or just not in the mood!

Feel free to gaze at the card illustration. Drink in the colors and imagery, and step through the portal to a mysterious and sacred world. Reciting the affirmation will also help you enter into the energy of the mudra.

You can use the deck solely for guidance without adopting the mudra postures. Alternatively, just flip randomly to a page in the guidebook and use the mudras you encounter.

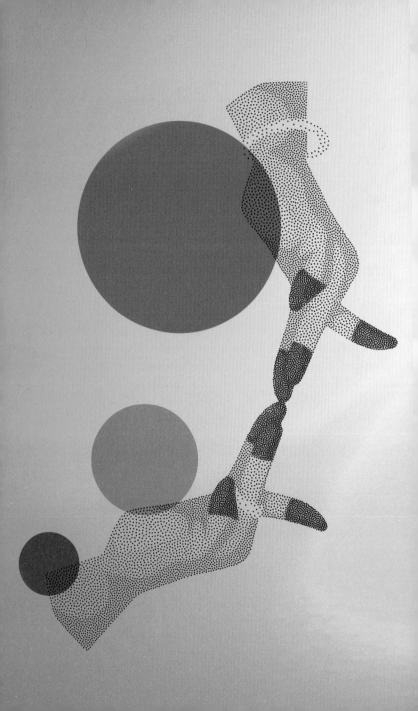

PREPARING, CLEANSING AND CONSULTING *YOGA MUDRA ORACLE*

How to prepare the deck

Touch each card one by one. Ensure you have a clear mind and heart, free of any fear. Shuffle the cards, then hold the full deck using both hands and perform the "regular cleansing ritual" outlined below.

This process is recommended both before you use your cards for the first time and anytime you feel they need an energy boost— e.g. you haven't used them for a while and wish to reconnect, or a borrower has returned them.

Regular cleansing ritual

Hold the full deck in both hands, taking three conscious breaths deep into the belly. Feel your energy bathing the deck in soft, white light. Infuse the cards with your essence—and everything you seek or aspire to—until you feel a warmth or slight tingling in your hands as the energy weaves through the deck.

You may wish to do this each time you use *Yoga Mudra Oracle*. But how often is entirely up to you.

Alternative
cleansing processes

Other ways to cleanse the deck include using one or more of the following tools, waving them over and around the deck:

- sacred bell/tuning fork/crystal bowl

- sacred smudging feather

- crystals

- incense

- ethically sourced palo santo or sage smudge stick

- something sacred of your own choosing

Remember, your intention is important. Sense the deck filling with light and love energy as you perform the ritual.

How to consult
Yoga Mudra Oracle
for yourself and others

In the spirit of experimentation with the deck and discovering what feels right for you, consider the following suggestions:

First, if cleansing is needed, hold the deck of cards and perform the ritual with a clear mind and a heart released from fear.

Shuffle the cards and cut the deck into three separate piles, laying the piles directly in front of you.

Collect all the cards back into one pile, then spread them out in a fan shape with one hand.

Select cards—with your eyes open or closed—using your non-dominant hand. Without thinking, draw the ones that call out to you. You may feel an energetic tingling as you hover over certain cards, suggesting they are meant for you.

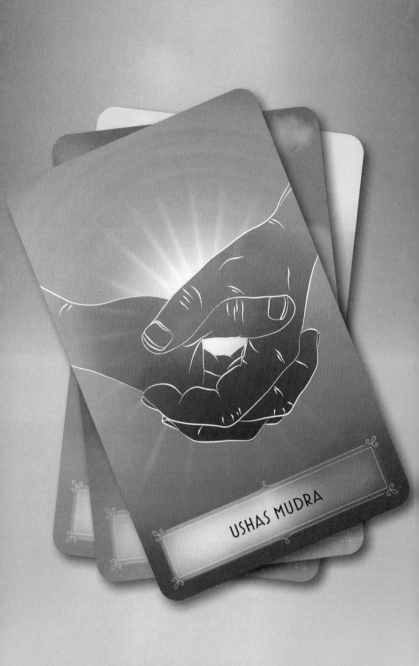

USHAS MUDRA

CARD LAYOUT OPTIONS

There are **four** card spread options for *Yoga Mudra Oracle* readings.

If your reading involves more than one card, move through the mudra poses one by one after reading each card's guidance. Try to feel and enter deeply into the card meanings, gazing at each illustration. Remember to take three conscious breaths while performing the mudra.

Take note of any feelings that might arise in you. Once you have finished your reading, you might like to try a mudra "flow"—that is, moving from one mudra to the next and again taking note of any impressions. If one mudra feels different or better than another, trust this feeling and perhaps work again with that mudra in your meditation or yoga practice.

Performing the mudras will help bring the card guidance to life. Meditation can help bring you into a space where you can explore mudras more deeply. You can find meditation exercises to support you here: www.emmawertheim.com

One-card reading

QUICK GUIDANCE:

Form a question. (For example: what would support me now, in this moment?) Draw one card. Reflect on the card message and mudra guidance in relation to your question.

Two-card spread

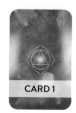 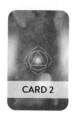

SOUL-CENTERED QUESTIONS:

Card one: What is my soul calling me to look at within myself right now?

Card two: What is my soul calling me to act on right now, to move forward in my life?

Three-card spread

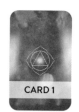 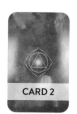 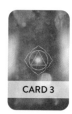

SPIRITUAL DIRECTION READING:

Card one: What has my soul or life journey been up to now?

Card two: What do I need to know right now, to move forwards in my soul or life journey?

Card three: Where am I headed in my soul or life journey?

Five-card spread

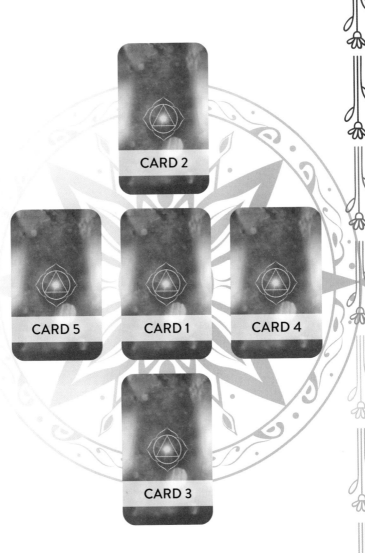

NODAL/LIFE PATH READING:

(Lay card one in the center of the spread with the other cards in a directional/ compass format around it.)

Card one: you. Indicates where you are right now in your life and the energies that surround you.

Card two: north. Shows where you are headed and the attributes you may need to develop to help you get there.

Card three: south. Indicates what you are moving away from or need to move away from and let go of.

Card four: east. Highlights thoughts and perceptions about yourself that may be hindering or helping you.

Card five: west. Represents your current emotional landscape.

With this more complex layout designed specifically for *Yoga Mudra Oracle*, you may, for example, feel the urge to focus on the "north" card in the spread (card one) and work with this mudra for an extended period—days, weeks or even months. It will help strengthen your life direction.

If one card resonates more than another, this may suggest a mudra that will support you on your journey. For example, if you are experiencing challenging emotions, you may wish to focus on the mudra that presents in the "west" (card five) position of the spread. Alternatively, if you are struggling to let go of something in your life, you may choose to concentrate on the mudra occupying the "south" position (card three).

There are many possibilities for working with the nodal/life path spread. Each time you work with this layout, focus on what feels right for you.

Jumping cards / cards pulled repeatedly

If a card falls out of the deck while you're shuffling or you keep drawing a particular card, take note! The Universe is guiding you. This mudra is important for your growth right now.

Again, if a card doesn't ring true, trust this feeling. Clear your mind and—from a place free of fear—choose another card.

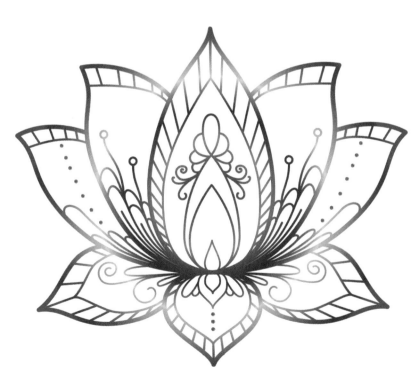

CHAKRAS

Some of the cards ask that you hold a mudra pose at a specific chakra (or energy center) in the body.

Chakra is the Sanskrit word meaning "wheel". In Indian traditional medicine (Ayurveda), yoga and meditation, seven main chakras are described, starting from the base of the spine and moving up to the crown of the head. Optimal health is achieved by ensuring these energy centers are in harmonious alignment, supporting the free flow of energy.

Please see the diagram below, which outlines where each of the chakras is located.

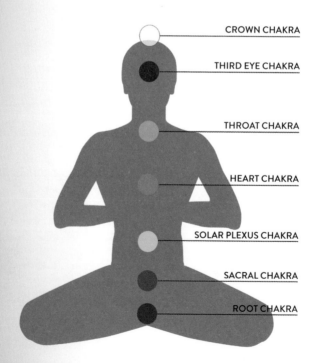

CROWN CHAKRA

THIRD EYE CHAKRA

THROAT CHAKRA

HEART CHAKRA

SOLAR PLEXUS CHAKRA

SACRAL CHAKRA

ROOT CHAKRA

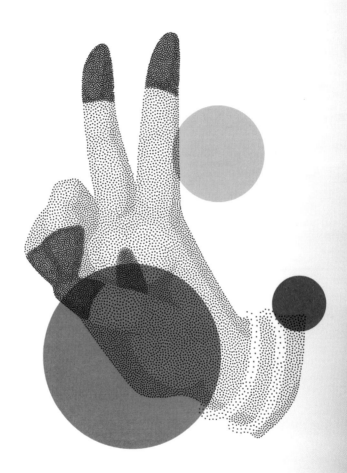

AND LASTLY...

While working with the deck, make sure you use the "stop" when coming to a conscious breath. The "stop" is an intentional pause between the inhale and the exhale of the breath. This "space" is where magic is birthed and grows.

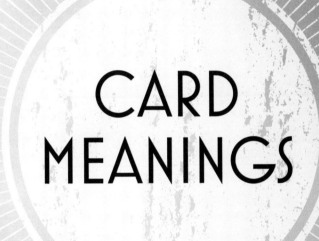

CARD MEANINGS

ABHAYA MUDRA

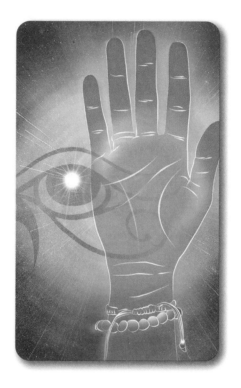

KEEP MOVING FORWARD

Courage, protection, clearing the path,
cutting ties, fearlessness, freedom.

You have the courage to take the next step on your soul path and life journey. *Abhaya mudra* will give you the strength and inner resolve to be true to your heart's calling—no matter what.

This card gives you the "thumbs up" to dream big and face any fears or doubts that bubble up. It asks you to examine any negative influences around you and break etheric energy ties to people who have let you down in the past. Send them love as you do so.

Abhaya is all about creating a new space of beginning. You may be delaying a project that could be fulfilling for you. This card is a reminder to simply make a start. Know you can move closer to achieving a major goal by taking that first baby step.

Being courageous does not always mean acting boldly or brashly. Courage can also ask you to hold back, breathe and step forwards from a new place.

Believe you can and will live a life aligned with your heart's deepest calling.

MUDRA

Raise your right hand perpendicular to your body, in front of your shoulder, palm facing forwards. Relax the hand, with fingers pointing upwards and shoulders relaxed. Imagine a warm glow radiating from the center of the palm of your raised hand.

Now rest your left hand in your lap (palm facing up when seated) or on your heart chakra. Or if standing, rest it by your side. Tune in to the quiet strength of this posture and let it dissolve any fears.

AFFIRM

With heartfelt courage, I gaze into the center of fear.
As it softens, my path reveals itself.

AKASHA MUDRA

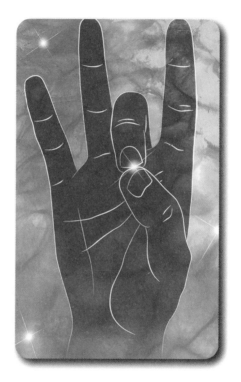

LIMITLESS POSSIBILITIES

Ether element, spring cleaning—
within and without, space, letting go.
Relieve feelings of heaviness,
live simply, give and share.

Akasha mudra helps alleviate physical heaviness and clear troubled feelings. Find a simple place within—a sacred void. It asks that you not fear the emptiness you may feel at this time. When we create space inside ourselves, we allow for the birthing of something miraculous.

You may also need to create space on a physical level. Do that long overdue spring clean. Donate anything that no longer serves you. Creating space in the material world around you will also cleanse and free you up on an etheric level, enhancing your spiritual well-being. You will feel lighter and more attuned to spirit.

Tune in to the fine vibrations of this subtle and multipurpose mudra. Allow for the void—a nothingness filled with potential. Limitless possibilities arise if you let go, release, and make space to usher in the new.

> *Among the great things which are found among us, the*
> *being of nothingness is the greatest.*
> — Leonardo da Vinci

MUDRA

Using both hands, bring the tips of each middle finger to its thumb. Let your other fingers relax as you rest the backs of your hands on your knees or thighs, palms facing up.

AFFIRM

I await, in simple garb, open and receptive—the
touch of the Divine upon my brow,
an ocean of love about me.

ANJALI MUDRA

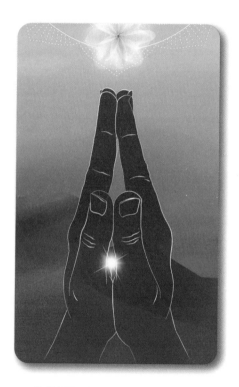

SOUL ALIGNMENT

*Saluting the divine nature of all beings,
connecting to your heart chakra.
Centers, balances and calms. Reverence,
devotion, surrender, humility, clarity.*

Your life is a soul journey. You are meant to be here. Know you make a positive difference to everything around you and everyone in your sphere of influence.

Just as a pebble dropped in a still lake causes ripples to radiate with the potential to reach the ocean, you have a vast and limitless ability to touch and transform the lives of others. In quietude and prayer, much is given. This energy is yours to emanate and grow.

Anjali mudra reminds you to incorporate more meditation and prayer into your life. Regardless of your religious beliefs, prayer sends a force of positivity into the atmosphere. It is an act of pure giving, tapping into an energy beyond ourselves.

This posture is steeped in mystery, possessed of great power for the good. But first, come back to your heart-space. From here, release pure and lifted intentions.

Hold a wish for yourself and others who share this magical life journey. Move ahead and travel well in the realization you are deeply loved.

MUDRA

Press the palms of the hands together in front of your heart chakra, with the fingers together, extending upwards. You might like to light a candle when working with *Anjali mudra* to strengthen your intent and seal your wishes. In both Eastern and Western spiritual cultures, this posture is one of prayer.

AFFIRM

My life is a sacred journey. I salute the Divine within myself and all beings.

APAN MUDRA

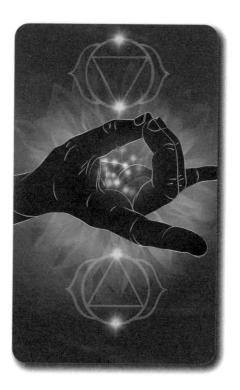

VISION UNFURLING

Springtime, new beginnings, balancing opposites, serenity, clear vision, energy, and removal of toxins.

With eyes of loving kindness, visualize your future self. You are invited to seed new beginnings in nutrient-rich soil, nourished by rain, kissed by the sun and blessed by the heavens. With gentle hands, tend to this reinvigorated, budding "you".

It is your time to nurture a harvest of purest potential. Allow the magic of this mudra to weave through your cells, presenting you with visions and feelings of who you are meant to be.

Fresh energy clears obstacles. But don't forget to have fun along the way. The destination is important, but the journey can be the real adventure.

MUDRA

Using both hands, bring your thumbs, middle and ring fingers together and extend the remaining fingers. As part of meditative practice, this mudra engenders a deep sense of peace. It is also a mudra used by practitioners when the liver and gallbladder functions need support.

AFFIRM

As my mind settles, I step into the garden of my heart, with the flower of new beginnings at its center.

BHAIRAVA MUDRA

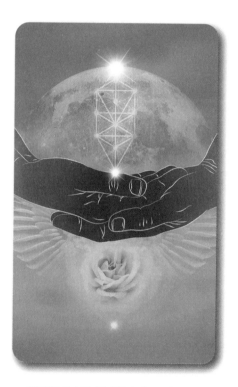

YOU ARE ENOUGH

A deity who destroys lower-nature negativity.
Promotes masculine energy and balances left and right
brain hemispheres. Releases ego and embraces life as it is.
Aids meditation, calming.

You are enough. In the face of challenging times or thoughts and fears of uncertainty, *Bhairava mudra* is a soothing balm, helping to dissolve negativity around or within you.

This card is asking you to be present—really and truly! A daily meditation practice can be a wonderful tool to infuse your day with positive vibrations, preparing you to meet whatever challenges come your way with a fierce peacefulness. Remember to "be" in this moment. It can change your whole life.

Simply open to the "now". All is as it should be. Slow down, even just a tiny bit. Be centered in pure presence. From this place, life will flow and move in extraordinary and mysterious ways, bringing joy and fulfillment. You are whole and complete.

MUDRA

Place the right hand on top of the left hand, with both palms facing up. Comfortably rest the mudra in your lap. Alternatively— to experience the feminine expression of this mudra (*Bhairavi*)— place your left palm on top of the right, both facing upwards. Take a deep belly breath and lengthen your spine.

AFFIRM

I walk the path of the mystics, well-worn by those before me. The sound of ancient bells echoes in sacred valleys, drawing me ever closer to soul remembering.

BHUCHARI MUDRA

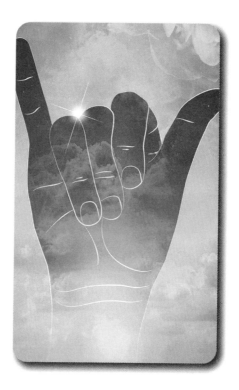

INNER SANCTUM

Sacred inner space, peace, expansion, clarity, rest.

Have you been feeling overwhelmed? *Bhuchari* calls you to turn your gaze inwards. To truly love, we must first love ourselves. It may feel counter-intuitive to take time for yourself when you are pulled in different directions. But if you have nothing left in the tank, nothing is possible.

This mudra asks you to enter and surrender to your sacred inner world. Fan the flame of peace that dwells there. Allow every part and aspect of yourself to be nurtured by the healing balm of quietude and timelessness.

In this place, you will be gifted an expansion of the heart and mind. Just as the clouds part and the warm rays of the sun touch your skin, so your every cell is replenished. From here, all is possible.

Take some time for yourself today. Immerse in your inner sanctum, and drink deeply from the well of your soul.

MUDRA

Using one hand, fold the index, middle and ring finger towards the palm, with your little finger stretched upwards. Bring your thumbnail to rest between your nose and upper lip.

Now gaze at the tip of the little finger while blinking as little as possible. Hold the posture for as long as is comfortable. If your eyes water, don't worry; this cleanses your tear ducts and sinuses. Remove glasses (if you wear them) before practising this mudra. Stay relaxed.

AFFIRM

I drink from the well of inner peace,
at the center of my being.

CHONMUKHA MUKHA MUDRA

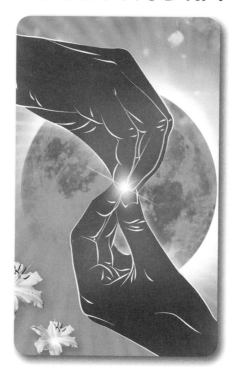

SOUL-CENTERED HEALING

*Attracting the right help. Balances solar and lunar
energies in the body and invites healing.*

You are exactly where you're meant to be in your life. If you are experiencing or have a history of ill health, you may already understand that important lessons and gems of insight can be garnered from times of challenge. In fact, these can facilitate change and expand your future, giving you greater understanding and compassion for others and leading you in exciting new directions.

This card asks you to be sensitive to your body and its needs right now. Make peace with your life journey so far. It has served a purpose. You may not understand it all yet, but, in time, clarity will come. Ask yourself, "What would support me today?" Whether the answer is loud and clear or just a whisper, listen to your intuition and be open to whatever form of support comes your way—including a doctor or professional who can provide exactly what you need at this point in your journey.

MUDRA

Use both hands. Gather the fingers of each hand together so all five pads of both sets of fingers touch each other. Start with your left hand on top. Bring both hands together so they touch at the fingertips. After holding this posture for a while, reverse the mudra so the right hand is on top. Hold the mudra in front of your solar plexus chakra.

To intensify the healing benefits of *Chonmukha Mukha*, touch the roof of your mouth with the tip of your tongue.

AFFIRM

*In the center I stand, as swirling patterns of mystery
fill my mind's eye, revealing synchronicity—
uncovering all that's been and all
that is becoming. Everything is as it is meant to be.
I am still.*

DHARMACHAKRA MUDRA

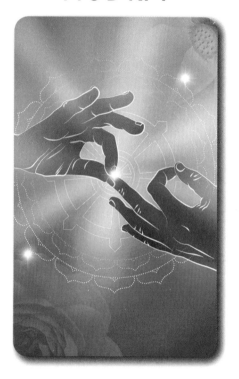

LIVING PRAYER

*Wheel of life (birth, death, rebirth and reincarnation).
Balancing inner and outer worlds. Change and
adaptability, trust and surrender.*

Make your earth body a living prayer, and keep faith in your heartfelt hopes and aspirations.

The unfolding of your life's purpose is close now. *Dharmachakra mudra* represents the moment Buddha received enlightenment—when his living vessel became a beacon of light and love and forever left an imprint of hope on planet Earth.

Prepare your earth self to receive and sustain a lifted energy of being that will touch all those around you and beyond. Make your body a living prayer, and know that this energy will attract all you have hoped and wished for.

The two hands in *Dharmachakra* posture symbolize "turning the wheel". In Hindu mythology, the wheel of life represents this life, past lives and reincarnation. The left middle finger, for instance, represents Saturn's energy, embodying karmic life lessons and uncovering deep mysteries.

Face old fears and forge a new path ahead. Accept this mysterious card today with grace.

MUDRA

Bring both hands up to your chest in front of your heart chakra, with the right hand higher than the left. Now bring your index finger and thumb together on each hand.

Turn your left-hand palm towards your heart and rotate your right hand so the back of the hand faces your chest. With the middle finger of your left hand, touch the point of connection between the right hand's index finger and thumb.

AFFIRM

My body is a living prayer. With each breath, I allow more and more light to guide my path. All is unfolding as it should. I surrender and trust in the great cosmic plan.

DHYANA MUDRA

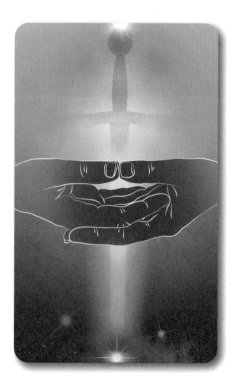

DIVINE DRISHTI

Drishti is Sanskrit for "focused gaze". Connection
to the Divine, meditation, releasing attachment.
Awakening, contemplation, renewal.

Do you recall a time in your life when the whole world possessed a magical sheen? Perhaps this was when you were a child. Or maybe later, you experienced a profound spiritual awakening or life-changing realization. Summon these recollections into your awareness today. The Universe asks you to open again to the magic delights and energies that flow through you and inspire your heart's true calling.

Whether you have a regular practice or not, *Dhyana mudra* asks you to let go of all expectations about meditation and give it a go. Simply stop and breathe deep into your belly. At the same time, visualize light entering through your crown chakra and travelling down to your root chakra. On the exhale, release any tension and negativity as you imagine the breath rising up through all your chakras, out the top of your head and beyond. Take a few breaths in this way. Be aware of your environment and allow for any noise or distraction. Let it all wash through you without attachment.

Gently focus on your breath again and place your hands in *Dhyana mudra*. As you breathe in, imagine you are an ancient oak tree with roots deep in the earth. Now feel your connection to the sky and stars as you exhale through your crown chakra.

MUDRA

Place your left hand in your lap, palm facing up. Rest the back of your right hand in the palm of your left hand. Bring the tips of the thumbs lightly together, forming a bowl shape.

Author's note: *Personally, I work with this mudra with the left hand on top, palm facing up. I feel it's a softer expression of the posture and feels more supportive in my meditation practice.*

AFFIRM

As chaos swirls about my being, I am the sword,
aligned and ready, waiting quietly in perfect balance.

GANESHA MUDRA

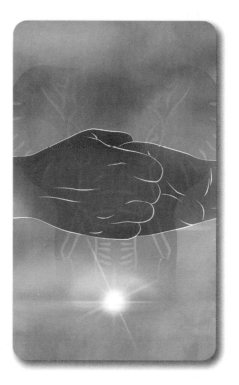

BREAKING DOWN BARRIERS

Ganesha—Hindu deity who conquers obstacles and opposition. Fire element. The elephant, representing courage and confidence. Strengthens the heart.

What is it that stands in your way right now? Is it part of your inner or outer world? Whatever this roadblock, this card is given to you now to remind you of your strength of character and inner fortitude. You have the power to break down these obstacles and move towards your goals—be they personal growth, fulfillment of a dream or your deepest heart wishes. At this moment, your heavenly guides gather to help you move through what may feel murky, towards a clearer picture of how to align yourself with your soul.

As we approach a dilemma, major life change or wall of resistance, things can feel extra challenging. Deep hurts may rise to the surface. Know that this discomfort is a sign you are cutting through old patterns, clearing away debris, and making space for light to dawn through the darkness.

Hold this image of the sunrise of a new day. Feel the stillness and peace. Work through old patterns of belief with a sense of new hope. Know that all will be revealed as you let go of old, fixed ways. Remember to call on the strength of Ganesha and your guides to be with you at this pivotal time of awakening.

MUDRA

With your left palm facing out and your right palm facing in towards you, bend the fingers so they interlock with each other in a grip. Hold for this a while, then repeat with your right hand facing out and your left hand facing in.

You might like to experiment with the following exercise: on the inhale, let go of tension; on the exhale, tense the grip of the mudra by pulling the hands apart without releasing them. Perform this mudra in front of the heart chakra.

AFFIRM

With Divine help and renewed inner strength, I cut away ancient patterns of belief to reveal a new day dawning.

GARUDA MUDRA

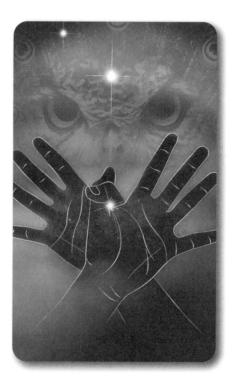

SHINE BRIGHT

*Garuda is the mystical, powerful bird that
Vishnu rides. Time to shine and be carried by love.
Helps with exhaustion and circulation and balances vata
(air energy in the body). Activates the solar plexus chakra.*

Don't hide your light under a bushel! Be bold. Be brave. Have faith and confidence in who you are. Voice your truth. Know you touch others in a profound way as you move through your life. You are greatly loved in this world and the higher realms.

This card carries a simple reminder—it's okay to take up space, speak your truth and be who you are. Yes, you are enough!

Some of us may think we have all the answers. But no one on this planet—not even the most enlightened of beings—has the full picture. Each one of us is a messy, beautiful, and divine work in progress.

Embrace all aspects of yourself. Go forth and shine your imperfect brilliance. Allow for the love around you to enter and fill you up. *Garuda mudra* will give you the confidence to do this. This healing force resolves opposition and allows you to move forwards with harmony and flow.

MUDRA

Place the right hand on top of the left and hook the right thumb around the left thumb knuckle. With the palms of the hands facing the body, stretch the fingers out like bird wings.

First, place the gesture in front of the lower two chakras (root and sacral chakra). Move it to the solar plexus and finally to the heart chakra.

AFFIRM

Soaring high upon wings of love, I see that I am enough. I have everything I need. I rise ever higher.

HAKINI MUDRA

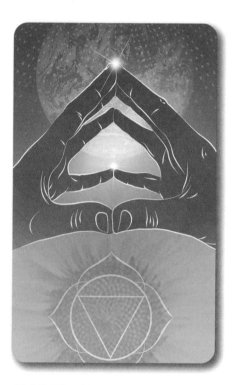

EARTH STAR WISDOM

Governs third eye chakra. Activates self-healing,
solves problems, accesses intuition, and boosts memory.
Focus, balance, clarity.

Author's note: *I'm always amazed at how many people perform this mudra in their day unwittingly. Start looking, and you will see it too. The body's intelligence is incredible—it knows what will support it!*

How can you create more space in your day for moments that nurture your heart and soul?

This mudra asks you to spend more time honouring your earth body and incorporating more healing practices into your day. This might mean meditating daily, moving your body more, having a bath, or finding a skilled reiki practitioner or massage therapist.

If you are required to focus on a project right now or you're in the middle of exams, *Hakini* will help you focus and access useful information for completing these tasks. It can also be used on the go for memory recall.

Performing this multipurpose mudra fosters harmony between the left and right hemispheres of the brain. It helps you feel centered and grounded and activates your body's self-healing powers.

Evoking the power of *Hakini* opens doors and allows energy to flow and shift, giving you permission to be kind and gentle to your body. In turn, this forges a connection with your eternal self.

MUDRA

Bring the tips of the left- and right-hand fingers to touch lightly. This posture is usually held in front of your heart chakra. But if it feels right for you, you might also like to try it in front of your third eye chakra. With eyes open or closed, direct your gaze or awareness towards that chakra. Relax your shoulders and imagine you are holding a sphere of light between your hands.

AFFIRM

Earth and star unite at my center, harmonizing and bathing my essence in love.

HAMSI MUDRA

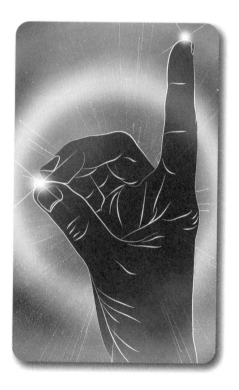

JOY

Playful, light, lithe of spirit.
Lifts depression and dissolves obstacles.

Allow joy to spark your life and touch those around you. The mundane and everyday can be a source of exhilaration, as much as life's peak experiences.

Even while washing the dishes, you can pause to reflect on the miracle of water and the playfulness of soap suds. Joy surrounds you each and every day. Seeing and feeling it is a matter of choice, not a lofty ideal. The more you tap into joy, the more it finds you.

If life has felt a little stale of late, you are called to remember happiness is a state of being—yours to be en-"joyed". When your schedule feels burdensome, carve out time for some "*joie de vivre*". *Hamsi mudra* gets you back in touch with childlike awe and wonder.

MUDRA

Approach this single-hand gesture with a childlike spirit. Bring the tips of the thumb, middle, ring and little finger together. Extend the index finger upwards. Hold it at a comfortable height.

AFFIRM

I remember JOY.
I make space for JOY.
I expand into JOY.
I merge with the bright spirit of JOY.

HAND-ON-HEART MUDRA

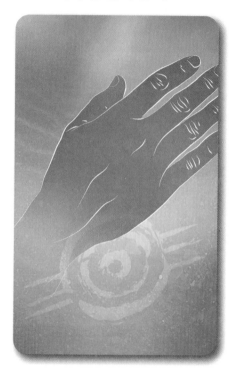

ANCESTRAL HEALING

Breaking free of negative family patterns.
Honouring your lineage.

This mudra has been intuited for the purpose of this deck.
It is a non-traditional mudra.

This card asks you to enter deeply into your origins, acknowledging the rainbow colors of your genetic history.

In many indigenous Australian traditions, paths that cross both land and sky are referred to as "songlines". Also known as "dreaming tracks", they are the routes travelled by ancestral creator-beings, connecting people with the land and sacred sites.

Similarly, our own ancestry lives within us like an ancient echo of living energetic pathways.

Visualize holding the hands of all your ancestors. See a chain of souls spanning all the way back, towards the center of creation. Focus on your heart energy, expanding to embrace these souls in a golden glow of peace and forgiveness—regardless of the sort of life they lived on Earth and the energetic resonance they passed down the line.

Let any tears or emotions flow and release them as they arise. Know that you are not the sum of this past story. You have an opportunity this lifetime to step free of your genetic conditioning, find your unique soul calling and share this beauty with everyone in your sphere of influence.

It only takes a single conscious breath to bring about a subtle change—an openness of heart and mind, allowing you to step on a new path and heal all those that have stepped before you.

MUDRA*

Place your dominant hand over your heart chakra and breathe deep into your heart-space.

AFFIRM

I honour and acknowledge my ancestral songlines, bathing my lineage in the golden light of the heavens and giving birth to my unique and sacred self.

HANDS-OVER-HEART MUDRA

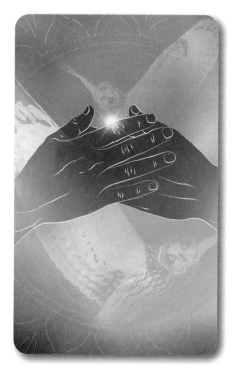

WINGS OF REMEMBERING

Attuning to spirit. Emergence.
Awakenings born of deepest insight.

*This mudra has been intuited for the purpose of this deck.
It is a non-traditional mudra.

This mudra prepares your being to respond to the call of mystery, the help that is uniquely yours at this stage of your journey. From challenge and profound seeing, now emerges a spiritual awakening.

This card reminds you that the trials of late shine a light on parts of you that need healing. You will emerge with new understanding and lessons that will never need to be repeated.

At such times, it's useful to remember the tools of divination at your disposal—this deck, meditation, and prayer. A pendulum, too, is a wonderful dowsing tool.

This card asks you to call upon your intuition and connect with Spirit. Listen to this silence within and allow your inner wisdom to light your path forwards. Learn to trust this space of connection. You are on the brink of leaving heavy karmic lessons behind you.

> *Life can only be understood backwards;*
> *but it must be lived forwards.*
> — Søren Kierkegaard

MUDRA*

With both hands placed over your heart chakra, come in touch with your breath. Send out a wish, asking the Universe for guidance. Let the higher realms and beings know you are open to receiving the help that is there, no matter what form it takes.

AFFIRM

I release my fear, and I open to guidance,
remembering my soul's purpose on
Earth as I emerge anew.

HRIDAYA MUDRA

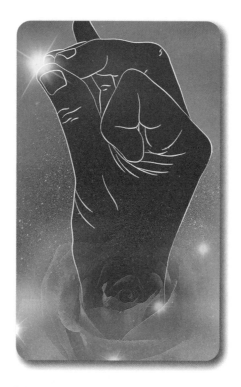

COMPASSIONATE HEART

Compassion, unconditional love, empathy, heart chakra.
Releases stuck emotions and assists with circulation
and respiratory issues.

Wherever you are now on your journey, view your life from a more loving, gentler, kinder place. *Hridaya mudra* helps you tune into your heart chakra. Take a moment to feel and enter this sacred space.

Imagine being a loving mother towards yourself and how this shift in point of view releases you from negative thought patterns about yourself. Bathe past actions and choices in the loving glow of understanding, and feel your heart released from their grip.

Use the energy of this posture to let go of emotions that no longer serve you. Open your being to love and peace. Let go of judgment of yourself and others.

Commune again with your heart. From here, all is possible.

MUDRA

Using both hands, fold each index finger downwards, resting the fingertip against the base of each thumb; the first knuckle of each index finger should press against the side of its thumb.

Now touch the tips of your middle and ring fingers against the pad of each thumb. Keep your little fingers extended but relaxed. **Please note:** *this is an intermediate mudra posture.*

AFFIRM

I breathe in the scent of the holy rose. I surrender and bathe in love. I envisage my life anew, with a gentle, compassionate gaze.

Author's note: *After working with this mudra for some time, I personally feel it is attuned with the energy of sacred feminine archetypes of compassion and unconditional love, including Isis of Egypt, Tara the mother of all Buddhas, and Mary the Madonna.*

JNANA MUDRA

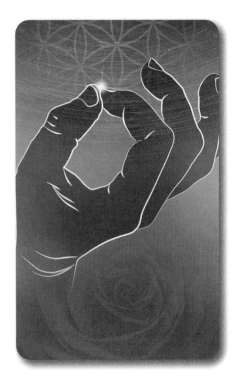

SACRED HEART SPACE

Heart-centered guidance, wisdom, intuitive knowledge.
Calms the mind, balances and connects to the Divine.

Hold a sense of sacred space and allow your heart to speak its truth. Light a candle, breathe deeply and quieten your mind. Let your heart flame expand out and touch the world with its unique color and healing radiance.

As you rest in quietude and inner reflection, allow words or visions to come to you. Be open to messages and remember that you are a being born of starlight. Through the portal of the heart, you can receive great and sacred wisdom.

Jnana mudra will help you open your sacred heart space.

MUDRA

Using both hands, lightly bring the tips of each thumb and index finger together. Now extend the other fingers, keeping the gesture relaxed and comfortable as you rest your hands on your thighs, palms facing upwards.

A recommended variation is to hold the right hand in front of your heart chakra (directed inwards and upwards) while the left hand rests on your thigh. This can be very stilling and evoke a feeling of oneness. Further, enhance this mudra by holding a clear quartz crystal in the palm of one or both hands and visualizing white energy.

This gesture is still used today in the Buddhist tradition.

AFFIRM

I allow for divine guidance, light and wisdom to open
as a rose within my sacred heart space.

KALESVARA MUDRA

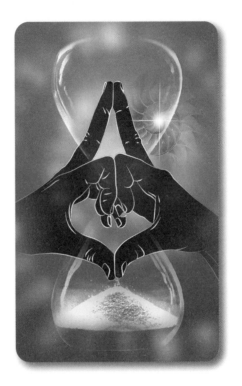

BREAKING OLD PATTERNS

The deity Kalesvara, who rules over time.
Breaks patterns or addictive habits,
calms the mind and settles agitation.

This complex gesture challenges your hidden aspects to rise to the surface, where they can receive the light of love. Becoming aware of negative patterns of behavior and addiction allows us to dissolve them. It's like turning a light switch on in a dark room. You realize there is nothing to be afraid of, as unwanted behaviors are bathed in the light of understanding.

The loving hands of this mudra reveal your true self and potential. As the famous Italian sculptor Michelangelo said, "Every block of stone has a statue inside it, and it is the task of the sculptor to discover it. I saw the angel in the marble and carved it until I set him free." As we confront the discomfort of unnecessary traits and overcome them, we grow as human beings. Be open to great guidance and courage from the Universe at this time. Step forward in love, shedding your fears.

MUDRA

First, press the finger pads of your middle fingers together, then curl your index, ring and little fingers inwards so their first and second joints touch. Bring the tips of the thumbs together, pointing these towards your chest while your elbows extend comfortably out to the side. The breath is key to unlocking the full potential of this mudra. While holding the posture, take slow deep breaths, focusing on the inhale and the exhale, sensing an opening in your crown chakra as you become more grounded. As your mind quietens, explore personal characteristics or habits you would like to let go of. Imagine transforming these parts of yourself. Ask the Universe for help.

Please note: *This is an intermediate to advanced mudra posture.*

AFFIRM

*With love and care, I open myself to release patterns
that hold me back.*

KALI MUDRA

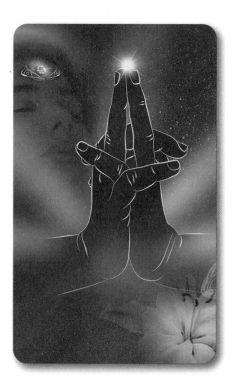

DISSOLVE ILLUSION

Kali is a Hindu goddess who governs time. Black goddess mudra. Pursues the highest truth and removes darkness. Groundedness, intuition, wisdom, inner fortitude, security.

Kali is a Hindu goddess who rules the fullness of time. She protects the innocent and destroys evil. Her fierce, feminine energy is a manifestation of Shakti, the mother of all living beings.

She visits your reading today to let you know your suffering is being creatively transformed. Alchemy is occurring within your very cells, even if you still feel stuck.

Understand the cosmic Law of Three, which applies to all phenomena on all scales, micro or macro. For every affirming force, there is opposition or denial. The reconciling—or third—force breaks the deadlock and allows for the birth of something new. This mudra helps you transition from doubt and fear to love and understanding. You will find your feet and foundation as this process reveals itself.

Kali's energy renews your faith and shows you a bigger picture. You will understand why your life hasn't been easy or straightforward. Looking back now with clarity, you perceive an intelligence at play.

Know the beings of light have your best interests at heart. They work for you and the greater good. You are supported and loved.

MUDRA

Bring both hands to your heart chakra. Interlock your little, middle and index fingers, ensuring that your right little finger is on the outside. Your ring fingers point upwards with both pads touching. Cross your left thumb over your right. Lift your elbows so your forearms are parallel to the ground.

Please note: *This is an intermediate mudra posture.*

AFFIRM

With grace and hope, I await the dissolving of illusion in sacred surrender to the unknown. I allow for a reality bathed in the sweetest vibration of love to open before me.

KUBERA MUDRA

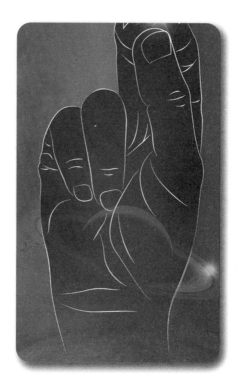

MANIFESTATION

God of wealth. Mars, Jupiter, Saturn.
Manifestation, initiation, intention, trust,
the Law of Attraction. Clears sinuses.

You are called to ACTION! Great change and opportunities are possible for you now. The answer to your question in your reading today is a universal, cosmic, earth-shaking, double-thumbs-up YES!

Kubera calls you to be in the space of openness. Here, you can consciously or unconsciously begin to manifest supportive changes in your life and respond to a yearning at your core.

Yes, you can allow for life as it comes and goes with the flow. But there is also a time to take life by the handlebars and set your course.

Nurture your sacred talents. Your natural gifts are your birthright, and they are meant to be shared. When you do, your whole being hums with creative energy, and expansive wonder fills your days.

Pray for guidance. Call out to your heavenly guides and be open to the help you receive with a fearless heart and committed mind. Harness the energy of *Kubera mudra* for manifesting things, small and large. Practice this mudra with a focused and clear intention and use it to achieve your life goals and fulfil your wishes.

MUDRA

On each hand, bring together the tips of the thumb, index and middle finger. Curl the other two fingers of each hand inwards, towards the middle of each palm. Place your hands on the backs of your thighs.

If your situation allows, speak your wishes out loud while practising the mudra.

AFFIRM

A rainbow of manifestation calls to me. I open the
door with a clear mind and heart and walk through.

KUNDALINI MUDRA

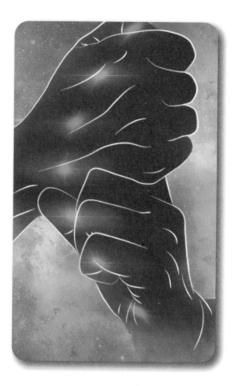

TRANSCENDENCE

*Root chakra, free-flowing energy, the union of opposites,
sensuality. Merging with cosmic consciousness.*

It's time to shift any stagnant energy residing in your lower centers. When our chakras are in balance, and our energy flows free, a door opens in our hearts, attuning us to the world of the soul.

Kundalini mudra helps you to harmonize and move through opposition. By accepting who you are now and where you're at in your life, you fast-track the transformation of negative self-beliefs.

You are invited to be you. Embrace your instinctive impulses and desires with love, acceptance, and forgiveness. Align with your higher chakras. Work with a conscious breath as you practice this mudra. When you are grounded and balanced, all your centers awaken, and you unite with your divine self. Shine now the rainbow colors of who you are becoming.

MUDRA

Form a soft fist with both hands. Extend your left index finger and place it into the right fist from underneath. The pad of your right thumb should gently touch the left index fingertip.

Now hold the mudra in front of your root chakra or as low as possible. The external world is denoted by the four fingers of the right hand holding the left index finger. The left index finger represents the mind and higher self. The divine world is symbolized by the thumb.

Remember to breathe, relax, and let *Kundalini mudra* work its magic.

AFFIRM

Naked, I am reborn in the realm of the soul. As my
chakras align, the colors of every aspect of my being begin
to harmonize. I am kissed by a warm, loving glow.

LINGA MUDRA

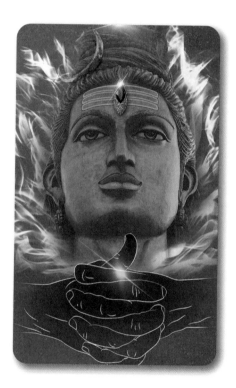

FIRE OF RESILIENCE

*Shiva, the god. Fire element. Removes toxins
and aids circulation. Warming, immunity.
Balances masculine and feminine energy.*

Spiritually speaking, this card is letting you know you are stronger than you think. Practice this mudra to bring heat into your body and cleanse yourself of impurities and toxins.

Visualize a fire burning away everything that no longer serves you—poor health, low self-esteem, negative patterns of thought or behavior. *Linga* helps you to build strength, clarity, and immunity and shore up resilience to face life with optimism, energy and zest.

This mudra is a sign you are being called to shift your perspective on your current situation. You are encouraged to see your life as the beautiful gift it is and move forwards with a new spring in your step.

MUDRA

Clasp both hands together and interlock your fingers. The right thumb should remain upright (masculine force). Encircle it with the thumb and index finger of your left hand (feminine force).

AFFIRM

The flame at my center burns bright and clear.
I am strong. I am powerful.

MAHATRIKA MUDRA

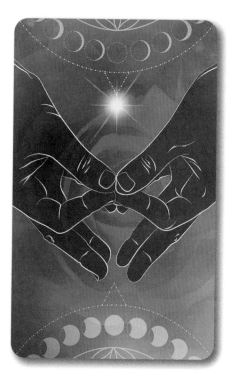

SACRED FEMININE

Mahatrika is Sanskrit for "great triangle".
Water element, sacral chakra, healthy emotions.
Assists fertility. Balances feminine energies.

Regardless of gender or how you identify, this card awakens the sacred feminine within and brings harmony and softness to your base centers. This is a time of deep emotional healing. The presence of *Mahatrika mudra* in your reading today assures you that a cellular rebalancing of vibration and energy is taking place in your body.

Mahatrika is calling you to release past hurts. Gently reflect on these memories and begin the process of understanding and transformation. Send loving kindness to yourself and others to seed the bud of new hope.

You are moving through a time of inner growth and learning. This knowledge will be of great help to you and others in future.

Honour this sacred moment when secrets are revealed. You are surrounded by angelic help as you bring tenderness and care to parts of yourself that need them. In your healing work, visualize a blossoming rose. Breathe in its fragrance and embrace this period of unearthing and awakening.

MUDRA

Starting with both thumbs and the tips of your index fingers touching each other, bring your hands together. Both little fingers should also touch at their tips. Relax the middle and ring fingers, keeping them straight but comfortable. This mudra points downwards. It resembles the shape of the pelvic bowl and should be held in front of your sacral chakra.

AFFIRM

*The rose scent of love cradles all of me in care and
tenderness. I breathe in its fragrance. I heal and release.*

MUKULA MUDRA

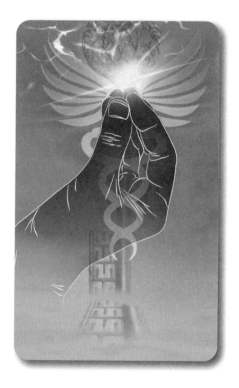

THE GOLDEN KEY

Focused energy of healing. "Physician, heal thyself."

A past trauma may have been unearthed recently. Or you may feel your body needs rest and care at this time. An aspect of your life needs addressing on a physical, emotional or spiritual level.

The key to healing past wounds or physical ailments lies within us all. Take a moment to contemplate what needs healing in your life right now.

To invite change on a deep soul level, allow healing to filter through your physical self and into your astral bodies.

If a physical ailment has been worrying you, use this mudra as part of the process of restoring harmony to your physical vessel and attracting the right support.

MUDRA

Purse all fingers of one hand together, then imagine your hand emanating a laser beam of healing energy. Gently place this beam over any chakra or part of your body that needs support. Now, do the same with the other hand and alternate from one to the other.

AFFIRM

I breathe in light on the inhale, welcoming peace and love. I release stuck, murky energy on the exhale. I invite healing into my being on all levels.

NAGA MUDRA

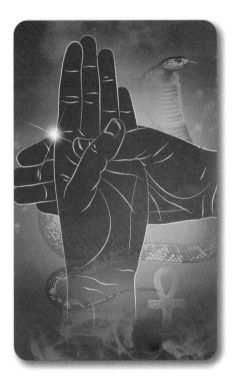

GODDESS RISING

Strength, intuitive wisdom, divine feminine, insight.
Solves problems and overcomes challenges.

The symbols used in this card—such as Naga (the snake goddess)—represent wisdom, fertility, and creative force. The ancient Egyptian *ankh* symbol is known as "the key of life". Fire represents the pure fire of insight and the awakening of potent energy within you.

This energy is rising through your chakras now, and the flame of insight is burning within you. Make time and space to embark on a journey unlocking what lies at the core of your deepest questions. Use *Naga mudra* and the exercise below to awaken your being to soul-centered wisdom.

MUDRA

With your left hand vertical, move the right hand horizontal and behind it, then cross your thumbs over each other—left thumb on top, palms facing towards you and in front of your heart chakra. Make sure you're comfortable enough to hold this position for a little while.

Sit straight and feel your breath deepen. Imagine a fire being kindled in your root chakra, with red (passion) and white (purification) or another color of your choosing.

Let the flames flicker upwards towards your heart and even higher, towards your mind. Sense a growing stillness within, then ask yourself a soul-centered question. Be open to receiving answers.

AFFIRM

The fire of insight burns bright within my centers,
opening my being to soul-centered questions and
answers. I hold the key to my awakening. I am ready
to receive.

NIRVANA MUDRA

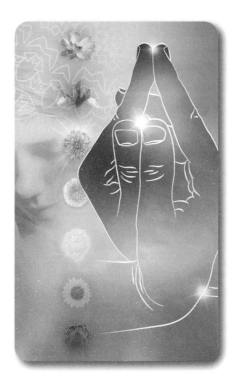

SIMPLE BLISS

*Freedom, awakening. Releases spiritual striving
born of ego. Used in rituals, dedicated to all beings.*

It is human nature to look forwards to happier times—when "this or that" falls into place. Often, there is a focus on material possessions or lofty spiritual ideals. But sometimes, only a simple shift in perspective is needed to realize that bliss and contentment are already there for you. Bliss is the birthright of everyone. It keeps everything in balance and allows us to live a full life, experiencing the color-filled gamut of earthly emotions. Loss and despair, love and joy represent two sides of the same coin. Both open our hearts in ways needed for healing and growth. Take a moment each day to be grateful for your life and its many gifts. *Nirvana mudra* helps you to release the "hard" energy of striving.

MUDRA

With left palm facing up and right palm facing down, move your right palm under the left. Now hook (tightly) the little, ring and middle fingers of each hand together (with the right little finger on the outside). Without letting go of your fingers, swivel your right wrist and arm in an upwards arc motion so your right hand draws up and over to the left side. Your fingers should still be interlocked, with the tips of your index fingers touching. The sides of your thumbs press together and face outwards.

Finally, bow your head and bring the tips of your index fingers to touch at your third eye chakra. This mudra is best practiced slowly, with reverence for yourself and all beings.

Please note: *This is an advanced and dynamic mudra pose and may not be suitable for everyone. You can try* Anjali mudra *("prayer pose") as an alternative, placing the gesture in front of your third eye chakra with your head bowed.*

AFFIRM

I breathe and align my centers. In humble gratitude, I acknowledge life's gifts. Thank you, thank you, thank you.

OPEN-PALMS MUDRA

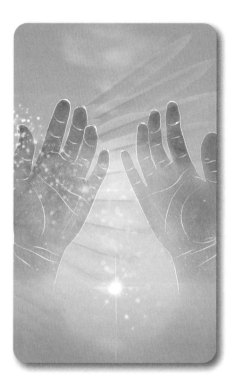

NEW BEGINNINGS

*Divine beings are supporting you. Prepare your body,
allow for new energy and be open to signs. Synchronicity.*

Something wonderful is about to happen for you. The timing of this might be unclear but know that great beings of light are weaving their magic, and your heartfelt hopes are about to become a reality.

This card asks you to prepare and open as you rest in tranquil inner reflection. On a physical level, you may need to declutter. Energetically cleanse your living space, allowing new energy to flow through your home. By creating space within or around you, you allow an invigorating "ocean breeze" to sweep through your life, inviting new beginnings on multiple levels.

Be alert to the workings of synchronicity at this time. This might take the form of physical signs or talismans of personal significance appearing repeatedly—like seeing a butterfly, a particular number, or a feather on the footpath. These can all herald that gifts are on the way for you. Watch for signs from beyond, reminding you to keep faith in your dreams. Exciting new beginnings are about to arrive.

MUDRA*

Place the backs of your hands on top of your thighs (or by your side if standing, palms facing forwards) and relax your fingers. Open your mind and body to the heavenly realms. Begin to feel a warm sensation growing in the center of each palm. Tune in to the sounds around you, breathe, and relax.

AFFIRM

New beginnings beckon. I make space within, expanding ever upwards, ever outwards. I fly through space and vast cosmic realms, beyond the boundaries of everything I am, towards all I am becoming.

* This mudra has been intuited for the purpose of this deck.
It is a non-traditional mudra.

OPEN-PALMS-TO-SKY MUDRA

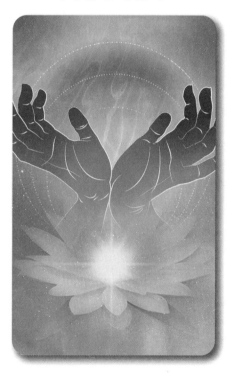

ALLOW FOR ANSWERS

Be open to guidance and allow for answers to come.

Perhaps something is troubling you right now, and you are uncertain about what direction to take or what your next step should be.

This card is about letting go and receiving guidance. By releasing your concerns and questions, you create a space where answers can come. Although it may not happen immediately, in time, it will become clear what you need to do. It is a gentle process that cannot be forced.

Trust in a higher intelligence. Allow for a deeper insight to rise up from the depths of your being and flower within your mind and heart.

Sit for a moment. Using the mudra posture, place your hands wherever the energy resonates the most—for example, in front of your heart chakra, high above your head towards the sky or moving through all your chakra centers.

Take deep cleansing breaths, release, and allow for answers to come.

MUDRA*

Open your hands in front of your heart chakra, and while breathing deeply into the belly, keep the base of your hands connected. Try raising your hands up towards the sky, then lower them back down through your chakras.

AFFIRM

*I let go; by releasing the question, I trust answers will
be delivered when I'm ready to receive them.*

* *This mudra has been intuited for the purpose of this deck.
It is a non-traditional mudra.*

PADMA MUDRA

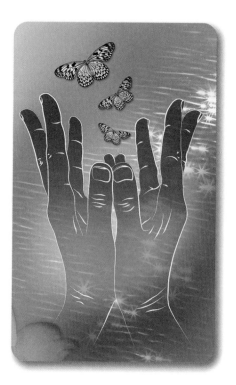

BUTTERFLY ALCHEMY

Opens the heart chakra and settles the mind.
Blossoming, releasing ego. Lotus flower,
devotion, love, rose quartz.

This card brings you the promise of deep healing and the realization of heartfelt wishes. It may herald that a new relationship is on the way. *Padma mudra* reminds you to connect to your heart, first and foremost. By finding more love for yourself and entering a space of vulnerability, you attract other souls of kindred vibration.

The lotus flower is a miracle of nature. Each evening it submerges into the murky water, roots grounded in mud. Every morning it re-emerges from the depths, blooming clean and pure, reborn in brilliance from suffering's muddy miasma.

A message is about to reveal itself to you. Open your heart to receive new insight and direction. Call upon your guides. Heed their whisperings and know this guidance is meant just for you. Right now.

Still your mind by taking a conscious breath and surrender yourself to the unknown—here, peace and love will greet you. You are ready to emerge anew and bloom in love.

MUDRA

Bring the bases of the hands together. Form an open flower shape by joining the sides of the thumb and the tips of your little fingers. Hold this mudra in front of your heart chakra and take slow, deep breaths. With eyelids half-closed, gaze softly into the center of the pose.

AFFIRM

I stand at the edge of the unknown. As clouds part and the sun's rays shine into my blossoming heart center, my spirit soars heavenwards, like butterflies released.

PRANA MUDRA

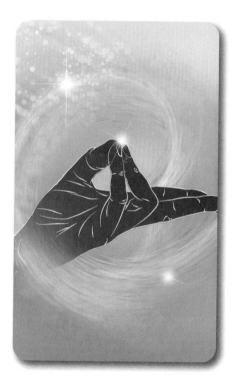

PRANIC FLOW

*Root chakra awakening. Destiny, vitality,
passion, amulets, activity.*

Believe in your higher purpose. Imagine and breathe in the scent of spring air imbued with the floral notes of nature. Awaken, invigorated with new life and vitality.

Gather strength from amulets. Keep a crystal in your pocket, place flowers around your home or wear a meaningful piece of jewellery. Use special objects to fortify and protect you as a reminder that an endless and abundant cosmic resource of energy is there for you. It is yours.

Harness the flow of your inner resources. Channel these gifts into areas where you wish to focus your unique and special offerings. You are about to enter a phase of your life where this influx of energy will fill and billow your sails.

This mudra connects with your root chakra, with the energy of Mother Earth or Gaia. Don't be afraid to activate this force within you. Allow it to flow ever upwards through all your chakras.

During this time of activity, motion and change, remember to do things that nurture you. Move more and find more time for things you love. Engage with people who light up your life. Act in harmony with pranic flow.

MUDRA

Using both hands, bring the tips of the thumbs, ring and little fingers together. Comfortably extend the middle and index fingers. Holding this posture, place the hands against the sides of the abdomen and relax the shoulders. Alternatively, place the hands on the thighs, palms facing up.

AFFIRM

Like a Sufi dancer, I spin and flow,
moved by the pulse of a cosmic heartbeat.

PRITHVI MUDRA

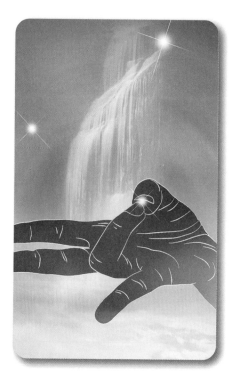

REPLENISH

Prithvi is Sanskrit for "Mother Earth". Inner balance,
groundedness. Activate root chakra, build strength, connect
with the earth, build vital energy and take time out.
Strengthens nails, skin, hair, and bones.

Replenish your vital energy. Reconnect with nature, drawing energy from her endless beauty. If you feel burnt out, insecure or out of balance, this mudra helps you to ground and renew yourself. Equilibrium will spiral outwards into your life.

This card suggests it's time to re-examine your schedule and carve out a bit more time for self-care and activities to help you relax and unwind.

Prithvi brings prana into your root chakra. It stimulates the liver and stomach. It connects you to Mother Earth, Gaia and her gifts—the beauty that surrounds you, the touch of sun on your skin, the sound of wind in the trees or the cleansing rain of renewal. It's time to stop and drink deeply from the sacred waters of the soul.

MUDRA

Using both hands, place the tips of each thumb and ring finger gently together. Extend the other fingers, keeping them relaxed. If seated, turn the mudra upside down so your inner wrists rest comfortably on the back of your thighs.

AFFIRM

I stand on the shore, touched by the mist of waterfalls,
kissed by Father Sun's rays and Mother Moon's glow.
I am held in cosmic mystery within a rainbow of hope.

PUSHPAPUTA MUDRA

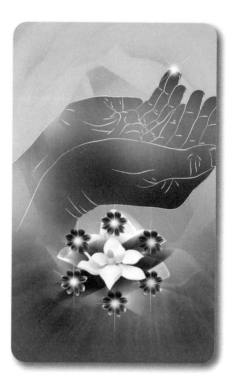

FLOWER OFFERING

*Giving and receiving, acceptance, openness,
patience and divine timing.*

Is there a connection between helping others fulfill their greatest potential and making your own dreams a reality? *Pushpaputa mudra* has entered your reading today, reminding you of a great esoteric principle—when you give with all your heart, you open yourself up to what may also be given to you.

When you see a flower, let it be a reminder to you: it opens selflessly and naturally in its own time. Nurture your seed of possibility for the benefit of all and leave the rest to divine timing.

Have faith that something special is about to blossom in your life. But first, know you are called to see beyond your own needs and concerns. Trust that the Universe has your back. Be patient. You are part of the sacred and divine order of all things.

In an open and quiet inner place, ask your higher self if it's time to act. Let go of your fearful, narrow self and its whisperings. Make space for a new way forwards. Put flowers on your altar or in a vase in your home as an offering to this sacred unfurling.

Let the natural world around you be your inspiration. Open and allow for divine unfolding.

Give, and you will receive.
— Luke 6:38

MUDRA

Place both hands in an open posture in your lap, like an empty bowl. The thumbs of each hand should touch the outer side of each index finger. Relax the hands and allow for a feeling of openness and acceptance to wash through you.

AFFIRM

I open to give; I open to receive. My hands full of flowers, I breathe deeply of their scent, transported to heavenly realms of possibility.

SAHASRARA MUDRA

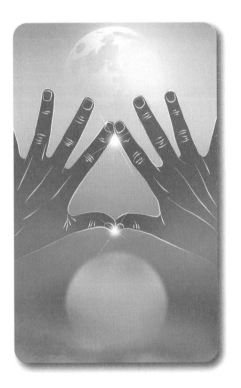

BE HERE NOW

*Thousand-petalled lotus, connection,
being in the moment.*

No matter what challenges you are facing right now, know this too shall pass. By taking a moment to lift your vibration through the taking of a simple, conscious breath, your perception can shift, and a new path forwards can reveal itself.

Stop. Breathe. Sense your whole body. Slow down and reset. Take a moment. Come in touch with pure sensation—the air on your skin, the sun warming your face, a tingling in your hands or the warmth of your heart.

Check in with your inner self to help you feel and be touched by all life. Calm your spirit. Deliver a mother's loving touch to your soul self. Connect more to the earth and nature's gifts—the majesty of the ocean, the viridescence of trees. Breathe in the rich scent of a rose, relish a mountain vista or birdsong.

Harness the energy of the sun, wind, and moonshine to ground and center yourself in your body. Embrace and make use of the tools of nature all around you to calm and embrace the oneness of all life.

MUDRA

Standing or seated, stretch out your fingers on both hands, palms facing away from you. Now bring your two hands together so the index fingers and thumbs touch, forming a diamond shape. Take *Sahasrara mudra* outside in daylight hours when the sun is not too strong. Hold the mudra overhead and feel the sun's rays warming your hands and radiating throughout your body.

You can also practice this mudra at night under the tranquil light of the moon and stars. Allow yourself to be healed head to toe. Experience the here and now, in contact with all life.

AFFIRM

I bathe in the light of the heavens and feel its healing touch. I am one with all.

SAMPUTA MUDRA

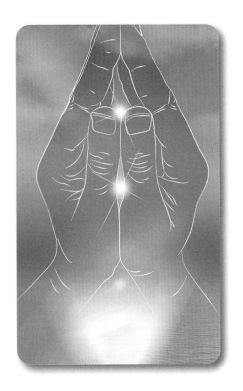

THIS PRECIOUS MOMENT

Bud of potential, equanimity.
Alleviates emotional and mental suffering.

Infuse this precious moment with your whole being. Release the past and let go of the future. Being here—right now—is all that matters. Persistent and gentle efforts to come back to the present enable you to surrender to this moment with an inner smile and gratitude for all you have been given in this life.

You may have not long ago lost someone dear to you. A shock is sometimes needed to awaken a renewed zest for life and a sense of purpose. This card asks you to remember someone who passed many years ago or just recently. Come in touch with their imprint of light in your heart. Let this remind you to live more fully in this precious moment. Treasure this person in your heart today.

To experience the fullness and beauty of this life, water the inner garden of your soul with conscious breath. Slow down and open your being to "now".

The *present* moment is truly a gift!

MUDRA

Bring both hands together, palm to palm, and create room between them where your thumbs can rest. Now direct your attention to this space between your hands, like you are holding a precious jewel. Hold the mudra in front of your heart chakra.

AFFIRM

I hold a bud of pure potential.
Within this precious moment— now.

SHANKH MUDRA

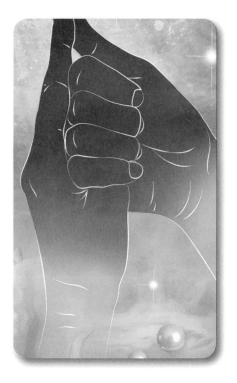

VOICE YOUR TRUTH

Throat chakra awakening.
"Om", conch shell, inner temple, color blue.
Supports kidney function and digestion.

This mudra is directed at your throat chakra, supporting you to come in touch with your heart's truth and speak it. It will help free something that stands in your way, an obstacle you are ready to lift and transform. Voicing your truth holds great power. Let go of fear and doubt. Know you can do it. The trepidation this brings up is less than you may expect. When you allow your true self to confront the situation in need of transformation, many doors of mystical manifestation will open for you.

Fear is simply a tool for growth. It can usher in new ways and a new being. Your soul is calling you to expand your understanding. Be bold and take a leap of faith. Free your voice and trust in the unfolding of a divine process guided by beings of light. You can use crystal singing bowls, a sacred bell, tuning forks and other tools to help open this chakra.

MUDRA

Wrap the four fingers of the right hand around your left thumb. Touch the right thumb pad to the pad of the middle finger on the left hand, forming the shape of a conch shell. Hold the mudra in the space between your heart and throat chakra.

Once the silence builds and a sense of peace deepens. Chant "Om" a few times. Let quietude envelop you. You may also like to meditate on the color blue and imagine hands of light pouring healing energy into your throat chakra. On the inhale, breathe in this light; on the exhale, release any feelings of "stuckness" in your throat chakra. From this place, you will find the courage to speak what rings true for you.

AFFIRM

I step into my inner temple, anointed by the waters of cosmic mystery. My throat is caressed by hands of love. Here my heart speaks its truth. I am heard, and loved.

SHANKHAVARTA MUDRA

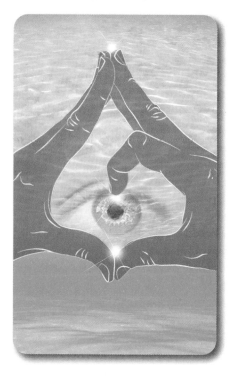

INTUITIVE SEEING

*Gateway to the heart. Access intuitive guidance
and calm the mind.*

Now is the time to quieten the chatter of your mind. Settle its constant questioning of your life and purpose—the "should haves" and "should nots"—and awaken the intelligence of your heart.

The breath holds the key to heightening the voice of intuition so it can sing and be heard. The pause between breaths is truly where this connection can be forged.

Try a simple *pranayama* practice called "square breathing". In a quiet space, breathe deep into the belly to the count of four. Hold there for another four counts. Then exhale for four and hold again for four. Repeat several times.

The quiet space you cultivate using this simple breathing practice will bring you whispers of deep wisdom as you dream. Over time you will recognize and trust this guidance more and more in your everyday life as flashes of insight seep into your waking consciousness.

This mudra deepens your connection to spirit, helping to align your chakras and awakening awe and reverence to the mystery and magic of your life journey so far.

MUDRA

Press the tips of all corresponding fingers together. With your thumbs extending downwards, bend the right index finger only, down at 90 degrees to the middle joint.

Honour this mudra as a portal to another world. Taking its shape opens you to new dimensions within yourself. Hold the mudra in front of your heart chakra.

AFFIRM

*From a quiet place within, I hear the pulse of the
Universe in the center of my being. My inner world
awakens; I am connected, one with all.*

SHUNYA MUDRA

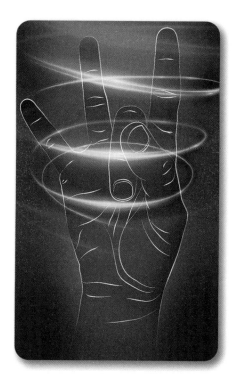

HUM OF THE UNIVERSE

Ether element. Open to divine truths.
Heaven, purification, forgiveness, quiet mind.
Helps earaches and issues with hearing.

Listen to the sounds around you. Tune into a deepening breath. Feel the breath awaken your body, and your cells awaken to an expanded sense of being.

In his book *Proof of Heaven: A Neurosurgeon's Journey into the Afterlife*, Eben Alexander describes an experience of leaving his body behind, with no distance between himself and "God", the "Mother" or "Creator".

Eben also refers to God as "Om"—a sound underlying all creation. "'Om" was the sound I remembered hearing associated with that omniscient, omnipotent, and unconditionally loving God,' he writes.

In Hindu scripture, "Om" is described as the original sound of creation, an aural resonance reminding us to get back in touch with the divine essence of all and everything.

Imagine this sound entering and expanding you. Listen to this "Om" with your whole being and body, not just your physical ears. Be receptive and open to what may come— visions, messages, the unlocking of old patterns calling you to forgive yourself and others.

You are ready to hear the deepest, divine truths. You may feel raw from this seeing. But vulnerability can be a strength—a sign of soul awakening, leading to deeper understanding.

MUDRA

Bend the middle finger towards the palm of your hand. Hold the finger in place with the pad of your thumb while you extend your other fingers upwards. Hold the mudra wherever it's comfortable. Practice using both hands.

AFFIRM

As my mind grows calm and quiet, I listen with my soul being, awakening to deep truths, ever expanding.

USHAS MUDRA

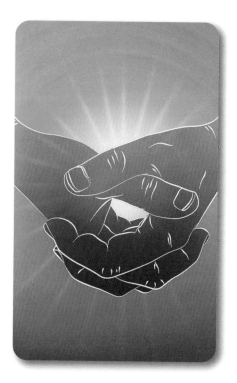

NEW DAWN

Sacral chakra. Unlocks secrets, balances hormones
and energizes and awakens creativity.
Colors of sunrise. Enjoy life.

On a new dawn, *Ushas mudra* beckons you to bask in the glow of daybreak. Imagine reds, yellows and oranges filtering through your body, touching and gently awakening every part of you.

You step into the spotlight on an empty stage. In this space, it is up to you to create the life you wish for, where deep peace is felt and vital energy restored. Know that your unique soul color inspires those around you.

Now is your time to hold space and accept everything you are. Know you are enough and much loved. It is time to enjoy all you have worked so hard for. Pause, be glad and enjoy.

MUDRA

Clasp the hands together with the fingers interlocked. For women, the left thumb rests on top. For men, it is the right thumb. Apply gentle pressure from the higher thumb to the lower one. Hold wherever it's comfortable. This mudra can be performed while meditating, walking, seated, lying down or standing.

AFFIRM

I accept all colors and shades within. Here, in this light-filled space, joy bubbles ever upwards. With childlike enthusiasm, I step the path that beckons.

UTTARABODHI MUDRA

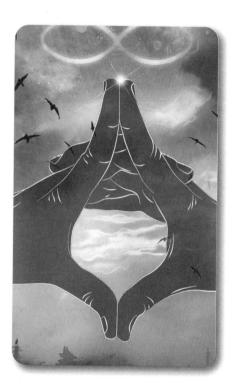

ATMAN AWAKENING

Atman means "the universal self" in Sanskrit.
Metal element, inspiration, motivation, self-realization,
soul enlightenment, calming, conductivity, energy.

If you've felt uninspired, low in energy or unfocused recently, this powerful mudra awakens and galvanizes. *Uttarabodhi* connects you to your eternal self, harnessing this relationship in support of action. Illumination comes to you on the wings of cosmic vibration.

This mudra strengthens your mind and has a fortifying and replenishing effect on your nervous system. It activates your inner reserves, bringing you clarity and answers.

> *Real love is a cosmic force which goes through us.*
> *If we crystallize it, it becomes the greatest*
> *power in the world.*
> — G.I. Gurdjieff

MUDRA

Using both hands, bring your thumbs and index finger pads together and interlock the remaining fingers. Hold this mudra in front of your solar plexus with your thumbs pointing downwards and your index fingers towards the ceiling. Hold the posture for any amount of time.

Please note: *this is an intermediate mudra posture.*

AFFIRM

I hold sacred space. Physical confines dissolve. My
spirit is set free, forever expanding in this precious
moment of conscious awakening.

VAJRA MUDRA

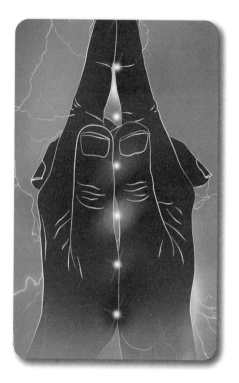

WILL OF STEEL

*Energy moving upwards to higher centers. Aligns chakras,
improves concentration, awakens and frees circulation.
Strength, thunderbolt, willpower.*

Do you feel you need more physical activity in your life? It's time to begin. Moving your body offers many benefits. *Vajra mudra* reminds you to make a start. No matter how small that first step, you will achieve immediate results.

Spiritually speaking, *Vajra* is urging you to act to clear any obstacles in your life, forging a new path. A bubble of the highest protection surrounds your body, aligning your chakra centers and creating an aura of unwavering power and resolve. You have the fortitude to face whatever is challenging you right now.

You possess an electric will of steel. Act from this place of conviction, aligned with a loving force.

MUDRA

Clasp your hands, index fingers extended and touching each other. Now bring the thumbs together gently with their pads against the sides of your two outstretched fingers. Hold this mudra above your crown chakra, with the index fingers pointing upwards.

Please note: *this is an intermediate mudra posture.*

AFFIRM

Amidst the crackle of thunder and the swirling winds of change, I stand in stillness, rain cleansing my body and spirit. Connected to my starry origins, I step forwards in love.

VAJRAPRADAMA MUDRA

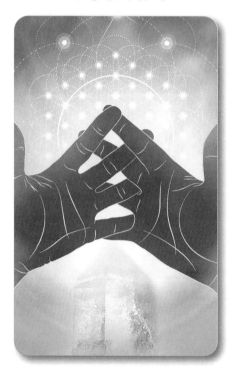

TRUST

Trust, fortification, confidence,
talisman, inner strength.

Vajrapradama mudra helps you release fears about the future. This card suggests you're at a crossroads and asks you to look at what is holding you back.

It's normal to experience doubt and insecurity in our lives. At other times, it is also not unusual to experience rock-solid conviction, as though a light illuminates the path ahead and the future is crystal clear.

When you truly see your fear, you realize it's often not as big or frightening as you originally pictured it.

Trust in something outside of yourself, connect to a higher intelligence and a bigger picture. *Vajrapradama* gives you the grit to step towards a more authentic expression of who you are and who you can be and are meant to become.

Allow this mudra to nourish and nurture your blossoming bud of potential.

MUDRA

Interlock the fingers of both hands, allowing for space between them. Hold this mudra in front of your heart chakra, palms facing towards you, relax and breathe. Allow for a growing sense of quiet and stillness to spread throughout your being.

It can be helpful to use a talisman while working with this mudra. Lay it near you or focus on it while you meditate. Channel the energy you feel into this symbol or amulet and carry it with you to remind you of your inner strength.

AFFIRM

In the quiet between each breath, I hold space for myself. Here the path is clear, and I release my fear. Here I allow for love and light to fill me up and guide me forwards.

VARADA MUDRA

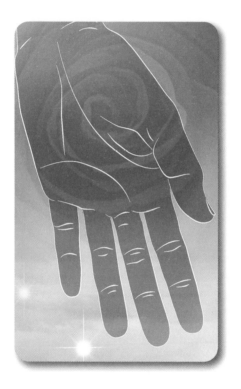

ROSE OF FORGIVENESS

Mudra of the gods. Mercy, wishes fulfilled and blessings.
Forgive yourself and others, accept, and heal.

A bounty of riches awaits the forgiveness of yourself and others. When you free someone of how they may have hurt you, you also release yourself. You can't change events of the past, but you can energetically change their imprint and hold upon you, allowing for a lightness of being. This opens you to a wealth of cosmic help.

Tread gently. Start small. To help shift these hurts, visualize a safe and sacred space, a glade or sphere of light. Bathe a person, thought pattern or trauma in healing light. Wish for their transformation, like a cosmic blue rose quietly unfurling. Come back to your heart center and give thanks for all that is good in your life.

MUDRA

In a posture of openness, open your left hand, palm facing up, and rest it on your left knee. Your hand should feel relaxed yet active, with fingers unfurled and tips pointing downwards. The right hand can either rest in your lap or on your right knee.

AFFIRM

Within the sacred glade of the heart, the blue rose of forgiveness blooms. Its holy scent is a blessing, a healing balm, anointing my centers with the oil of transformation.

VARUNA MUDRA

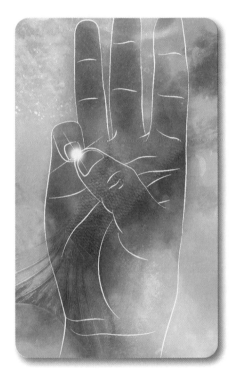

FLOW IN SPIRIT

Water element, guardian of the oceans.
Cooling, rejuvenating, invites flow. Innovation, energy.
Refocuses life goals and relieves congestion. Beauty.

This mudra asks you to connect with the element of water. Come in touch with the ebb and flow of life and its natural cycles. It's time to retreat, replenish, and draw energy from the ocean. *Varuna* urges you to examine where you are at in your life and drop your resistance.

Sometimes you just need to "go with the flow"; trust and set your sail towards the unknown, allowing things to open up naturally. Don't force matters; let it happen. If you're working towards something important in your life, this mudra asks you to trust that what comes is meant to be.

Support is gathering around you now for a most favourable outcome, one you would never have thought possible. And yet, most deserved. Stop, connect to your intuition and be guided by it.

Be like the mountain stream, continually adapting and changing as you flow towards a great ocean brimming with life.

Mystical energy enters your reading today. Reflect, reconnect, stop, and collect yourself before taking the next step.

MUDRA

On both hands, bring the thumbs and tips of the little fingers together and extend the other fingers. Rest the backs of the hands on your thighs, keeping the gesture relaxed. Focus on the intention of this mudra.

Please note: *avoid taking this mudra posture if you suffer from water retention.*

AFFIRM

Bathed by a cleansing waterfall, I ask myself what must I let go of and how might I change? I allow for the whisper of guidance and wait for its unfolding.

VISHNU MUDRA

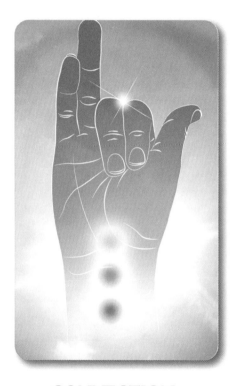

CONNECTION

Ancient Indian God: protector of the world.
Balances the lower chakras, aligns physical and
energetic bodies, releases stress and calms emotions.
Equilibrium, purification, grounding.

If you've struggled recently to feel the light in your life, be not afraid to enter that darkness. It is fertile ground, a necessary precursor of illumination. *Vishnu mudra* helps you transition through difficult times towards a truer connection with your soul.

Trust that the stars are aligning for you. This mudra lets you know you are safe and protected. All is as it should be. The heavenly wheels turn in your favour. You stand at the brink of a new chapter, learning how to balance both sides of your earth nature.

Let Vishnu take your hand and lead you towards true connection.

MUDRA

Use your right hand only, even if your left hand is dominant. Bend the index and middle fingers towards the palm of this hand. Keep your thumb, ring and little finger extended. Place your hand wherever it's comfortable.

AFFIRM

Held in a moment of stillness, the balance of night awakening to day, I move towards my destiny, connected to a higher intelligence. I am embraced within a sphere of love and protection.

ABOUT THE AUTHOR AND ARTISTS

EMMA WERTHEIM— AUTHOR AND ARTIST

Emma is a Sydney-based meditation, yoga and sacred dance teacher with a special interest in yoga mudras. She is also a graphic designer, intuitive digital artist and photographer. Her work conveys a sense of peace and hope, reminding us that the ebb and flow of mystery is woven through everyday life. Her art has been featured on book covers, websites, greeting cards and oracle decks.

She has been part of a spiritual school since 1995, which evolved out of the Fourth Way movement. Today this school's teaching is dedicated to growing moments of stillness as the basis of transformation, to walk a soul path in everyday life.

Birthing *Yoga Mudra Oracle* has been her long-time vision. In collaboration with husband and writer/artist Steve Denham, it is the culmination of a wish to share and communicate the simple ancient wisdom and the multi-dimensional benefits of yoga mudra hand gestures.

Instagram: @emmawertheim_
Facebook: emmawertheim.mudras
Website: www.emmawertheim.com

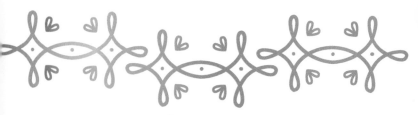

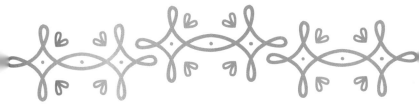

STEVE DENHAM— ARTIST AND EDITOR

From the age of nine, Steve's heart has always answered the call of the creative arts. He is a published author and freelance writer and has been shortlisted for several major Australian poetry prizes.

Steve's long-standing daily practice of meditation and breath awareness has flourished within a spiritual community in Sydney's north. This Fourth Way school is dedicated to cultivating stillness in everyday life, as the basis of transformation and realizing soul potential.

Instagram: @the_noholdsbard

Website: www.stevedenham.com

Art: www.bluethumb.com.au/steve-denham

Acknowledgements

Thank you, Steve, my dear heart-soul collaborator. Without your artistic gifts and 'next-level' writing/editing skills, this magical creation would simply not have been possible.

Family and friends—your encouragement means everything to us. Thank you to Jules Sutherland, Peter Loupelis and Sophie Macintyre for their excellent editing work. And to the wonderful Tania Ó Donnell and the Publishing team at Arcturus, we extend our deepest heartfelt thanks for your support and belief in *Yoga Mudra Oracle*.

Resources

The resources below were invaluable in my research into mudras and their healing and spiritual benefits. If you are interested in delving deeper, they are highly recommended.

Mudras: Yoga in your Hands—Gertrud Hirschi, Coronet Books

Mudras for Modern Living—Swami Saradananda, Watkins Publishing

Mudras of Yoga—Cain Carroll with Revital Carroll, Singing Dragon

Connect with us

We would love to hear how you work with *Yoga Mudra Oracle*. Share your journey:

Instagram: @emmawertheim_ & @arcturusbooks
Facebook: emmawertheim.mudras
Website: www.emmawertheim.com—for updates and inspiration
#yogamudraoracle #arcturusbooks

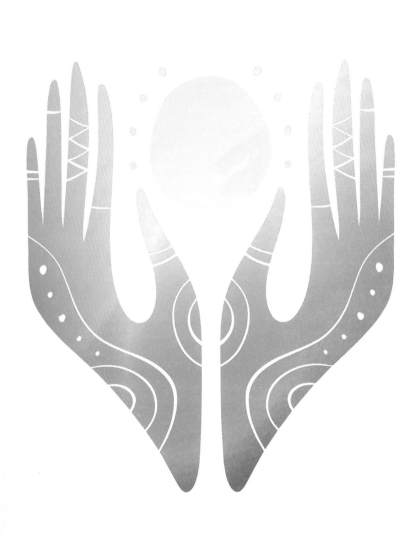

INDEX

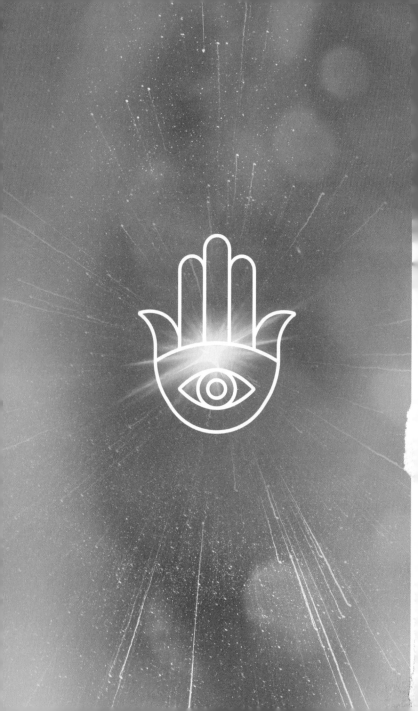